M.D. *Or* N.D.
What Should I Be?

How To Choose Between Conventional And Alternative Medicine As A Career.

By Dr. Christopher Maloney, N.D.

Christopher Maloney, N.D.

DEDICATION

To all those who wander, but are not lost.

And to those that wander, are lost, and still
find their way home.

CONTENTS

ACKNOWLEDGMENTS

I owe a great debt to my family, my teachers, and the wonderful students at NCNM. Thank you all for helping me with my decision, and supporting me in its fruition.

DISCLAIMER

The following contains emails sent to me over ten years. Many have been very similar. To protect the identity of those sending the emails I have deleted any identifying information. Any similarity to anyone you know is very likely to be coincidence.

I'd like to think that the same people who read standard medical disclaimers in self-help books will realize that it goes triple for medical decision making books. The purpose of this book is to give you information for an informed decision, not to make it for you.

My local hospital corrects my
N.D. degree to an M.D. My
profession is considered a typo.

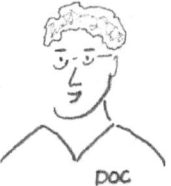

CHAPTER ONE: AN OFFER

When I graduated from NCNM many years ago and moved to Maine, I basically went insane painting my house and studying for my licensing boards at the same time. Then suddenly I had about a three month window between passing boards and being officially licensed. So I learned basic website making from a template and found a blog of Naturopathic questions without anyone answering them. Since I didn't have a lot to do, I started to answer questions. I have answered several hundred questions over the years, but none has generated more email than one response I did back in 2002.

On the forum, the sections are defined in various ways, one of which is a section on Naturopathic education. Curious students write in about various questions, including the major decision of whether to pursue a Naturopathic degree or a degree in conventional medicine. It is a clear indication of their confusion that they would put any weight on the opinions of strangers writing in an anonymous forum.

In response to one request for opinions about the matter, I wrote the following:

"Re: ND vs. MD

I was almost on my way to regular medical school when my good friend (Harvard/Brigham and Womens) took me aside and told me that what he was doing was killing him and that I should get out. I strongly suggest reading JAMA's survey articles on residency. Another close friend said that the public sees doctors like the actors on ER while the doctors themselves know the reality is like Scrubs.

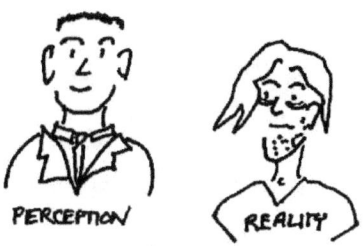

Being an ND is like any alternative to the mainstream, everyone gets lumped together (think Green party). So while I practice review article, evidence-based medicine, my fellow ND may only be doing Polynesian hymn bodywork.

The truth is the vast majority of the population simply doesn't know we exist. If you've even found this website, chances are your pull is a strong one. Please write me at docleroymaloney@hotmail.com, and I'll send you a letter I wrote myself for every time I wish I'd gone to regular medical school. Oh, and if you decide to go MD, apply to U of Arizona and do Dr. Weil's program.[i]""

Since posting that comment, which now is part of a hard-to-reach archive, I've received hundreds of requests for the letter I wrote to myself. After getting a couple more requests this past week, I realized that no one is addressing the question of how and why to choose an alternative medicine path. If my poor little comment is still in demand a decade later, it's time to write a bit more about the complexities of choosing alternative medicine. Even those with courage enough to write to me rarely ask for the information they really want: how do I make a decision?

Here's a short quiz.

M.D. Or N.D.

On a scale of one to ten (one not important and ten very important) rate yourself on the following questions:

1. How important is respect to you?
2. How important is money to you?
3. How important are your coworkers compared to you clients?
4. How important is it that you receive a regular, predictable salary?
5. How important are the M.D.s in your family?
6. How much do you like technology?

The higher your overall score, the less likely you are to do well as an N.D.

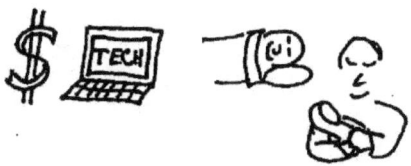

Here's another quiz.

1. How important is a good night's sleep to you?

2. How important are healthy habits to you?

3. How important is it for you to love everything that you do?

4. How important is family time in your life?

5. How important is it for you to have control over your schedule?

6. How important is it for you to have a low stress work environment?

The higher your score, the less likely it is that you will do well as an M.D.

How did you score?

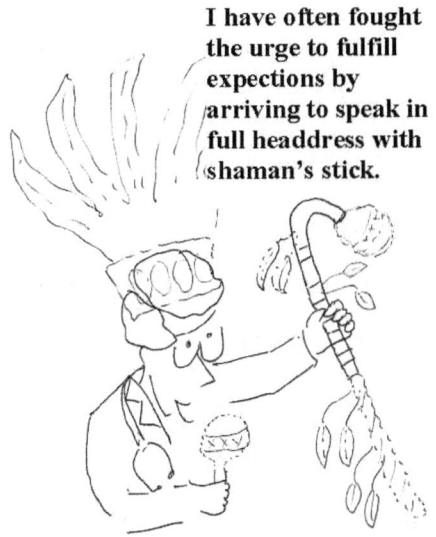

I have often fought
the urge to fulfill
expections by
arriving to speak in
full headdress with
shaman's stick.

CHAPTER TWO: THE LETTER

It is important to note that we talk differently to different people. Much of what follows is based on correspondence with individuals and largely a discussion of the problems and difficulties faced within either profession.

I am, of course, a Naturopathic Doctor, so it would be an error not to take everything I say with a pinch of potassium (or organic sea salt, if you must). I have practitioners in every field that I love and have the highest esteem for. But a discussion of their many, many great qualities would do little to aid a prospective student in making a decision. It is ultimately your awareness of the dirt, the difficulties, and the hurdles that need to be overcome that will determine your success in any field.

Also keep in mind that I have written to individuals over the years. Some began their discussions with attacks on alternative medicine, some with derisive comments about MDs. If you are offended by what appears here, keep in mind that we were writing to each other in context. I have preserved much of our discussions intact because many of you would not feel comfortable asking me such blunt questions, but will benefit from the answers.

The Responses, a Sampling of Quotes

"I hope you don't find this strange but I nabbed your email from a ND advice forum and was hoping you wouldn't mind giving me some advice as a practicing ND."

"I never knew there was such a thing called Naturopathic Medicine."

"You posted that you had written a letter to yourself every time you wished you had gone to conventional medical school. I'm wondering if you might share that with me."

"You said on this thread that you wrote a letter to yourself, do you still stand by it?"

"Is a copy of your letter to yourself about why you chose Naturopathic medicine still available and may I have a copy?"

"Why is it that you recommend MD over the ND program?"

"It would be great if you can send me the letter that you wrote for every time you wished that you had gone to regular medical school."

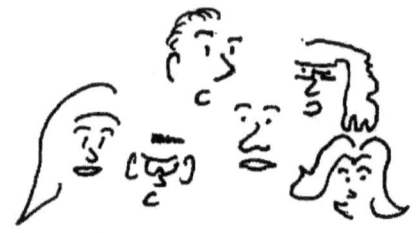

The Letter I Wrote Myself

Here's the original letter I wrote myself to dissuade myself from regretting not going to "regular" medical school. It says almost nothing about alternative medicine, and is based on the negative facts of conventional medical practice. I wrote it to give me a boost every time I faced prejudice, every time I dealt with contempt, and every time I worried about income while watching my conventional colleagues drive new cars. It shored up my resolve that for me and my young family I had made the right decision.

Since this letter and much of the rest of this book will talk about the problems with choosing an M.D. path, let me take a few moments to repeat what the vast majority of people will tell you about your decision: "Are you nuts?

Your aunt/cousin/neighbor/parents continue: "Of course you want to become an M.D. and not that whatever-it-is! Becoming an M.D. is the safest way for you to have a good life and take care of your family. You're so smart, and so dedicated. Don't waste your time thinking about any other field. Let's get those twenty medical school applications going, shall we?"

Christopher Maloney, N.D.

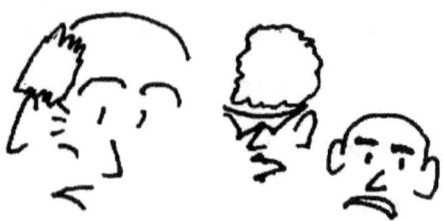

If you need more of the above, simply ask any of your relatives and pretty much anyone over fifty. Good, now we've heard that side of the discussion.

The situation described in this letter has not improved in the last ten years. Despite federal laws requiring limitations on residency hours, residents inform me that they are expected to cover shifts that exceed legal limits. At the same time medical students are expected to pick up the slack, and average one-hundred-and-twenty hours a week in hospital shifts. Please contact your local medical students and ask about their schedules and lives for a frank confirmation of what is written below.

"Dear Would Be Doctor:

Soon you may enter the medical field.
Your friends and family are in awe. Such a
great field, and you're so noble for wishing
to enter it. You'll be helping people. And
you can be sure that, as a doctor, you'll have
a successful life. Perhaps you should read
The Medical Marriage, by Wayne and Mary
Sotile, published in 2000 by the American
Medical Association. The book is
promedicine, it just gives a better
understanding of what you and your family
may experience.

Your career:

More than 50% of practicing physicians
say they would currently discourage future
generations from entering their profession.
(All cites are taken from the book. This is
from page 3. Remember, the book was
published by the AMA. Its facts are pretty
reliable.)

Approximately 80% of medical students reported being verbally attacked, and 24% claimed to have been physically abused during their training. This did not include the sleep deprivation, with wakeful periods ranging from 30 to 100 hours at a time. 81% of women physicians in training reported being sexually harassed or mistreated by clinical faculty or their superiors, and 50% of Latino students suffered racial harassment or discrimination. (p.23)

Research from England, Denmark, Scotland and North America shows that physicians and their spouses have increased incidences of drug abuse, alcoholism, depression, thoughts of suicide, acts of suicide, and psychiatric hospitalizations. (p.3) The suicide rate is twice that of the general population. (p.49)

Approximately 40% of female and 27% of male medical students experience pronounced symptoms of anxiety and depression. Compared to controls, medical students are five and a half times more likely to use sleeping pills, stimulants, and other drugs. The pressure is intense, and actually increases upon graduation. Worldwide research indicates that the rate of drug dependence for physicians is somewhere between 30 and 100 times greater than for the general population. (p.18)

The all-cause mortality rates of physicians are higher than those for all other professionals combined. (p.19)

While the average woman lives ten years longer than the average man, the average female physician lives ten years less than the average male physician. (p.19)

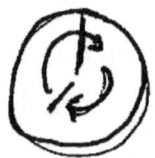 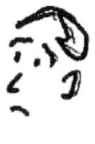

The average male physician works between 68 and 80 hours a week. The average female physician works 90% of this amount, while covering almost all home duties. (p.24)

Your home life:

Physicians under 45 indicated their major stress was the struggle with work/family imbalance and home life. (p.3)

Physicians tend to divorce less, but be less happy in their marriages. (p.4)

Approximately 50% of first time marriages of the population under 35 end in divorce. (p.3) Women physicians are 40% more likely to divorce than their male colleagues. (p.5)

Partners in a medical marriage tend to cooperate in normalizing a lifestyle that sanctifies workaholism, competitiveness, controlling behavior, doing and thinking too many things at once, and generally living in a self-focused haze of hurry sickness called super couple syndrome.

75% of physician spouses expected stress to decrease after residency, but 50% reported that stress actually increased after residency. (p.28)

When male physicians become parents, they increase their hours of work. (p.38)

You:

Most high-powered people deny that all of the above applies to them. (p.29)

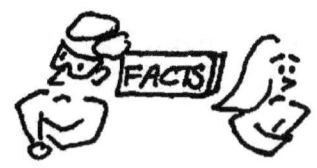

After more than a decade, I can assert with clarity that the book does not lie. I have seen too much pain among some of our finest doctors.

Here is some of the most recent data on gender inequality.

Christopher Maloney, N.D.

"Women remain underrepresented in PD (program director) appointments relative to the proportion of female medical school faculty and female residents.[ii]"

"There is a high incidence of sexual harassment and gender discrimination in academic health center (AHC) settings according to multiple surveys of medical students… describe their complaint process, components of their prevention training, and the outcomes of 115 complaints. (My note: Keep in mind that every documented complaint jeopardized or destroyed the career of that "complainer.")[iii]

My closest friends who are conventional doctors have been pushed in inhuman ways and experience ongoing stresses that would make them advise their patients to quit their jobs for health reasons and never look back. These are some of the brightest, sweetest, and most dedicated people I know. It troubles me greatly to see them striving so hard and receiving nothing but complaints from their administration and their patients. The phrase: "No good deed goes unpunished" seems unfortunately true.

Take some time to write down your reactions to my letter. Assume everything I say is false, then true.

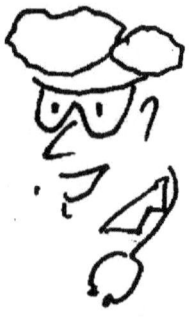

I wanted to be a vet, but humans bite less often!

CHAPTER THREE: APPLES AND ORANGES

As I get farther away from school, I am flabbergasted that I spent so much time thrashing about with the decision of conventional vs. alternative medicine.

Imagine two doors. Behind the first is a complex wilderness, full of plants but almost empty and with many unknowns. You will need to be self-sufficient and the care you give will be limited to what you can provide. Your life and time are entirely your own. Beyond survival, you are free to explore anywhere, do anything. But there are few clear trails, and much of what you do will need to be created from scratch.

Behind the second door is a vast machine. Hundreds of thousands of workers support complex technological marvels. Each individual is a cog, and the complex functioning of the machine is dependent on each person doing his/her own part. You are a vital cog, and your ability to perform the required tasks will determine the success or failure of your group's interaction with a patient. The time you have will be at a premium, and your ability to manage the dozens of tasks demanding your time will directly impact the amount of sleep and leisure time you have available.

The concept that there is any comparison between the two fields is a delusion. Both happen to address roughly the same health issues, but within an entirely different framework. It's like comparing becoming a trapper with becoming a textile mill manager because both careers roughly address the concept of clothing. To make the conceptual difference clearer, I provide a pro/con list in the style of Benjamin Franklin.

The Pro/Con List

We are talking about choosing between two very different careers.

MD: Patients consider you Godlike.

ND: Patients consider if you are a fraud.

Even after becoming an N.D., I want to believe my M.D. has godlike abilities. This is a two-edged sword.

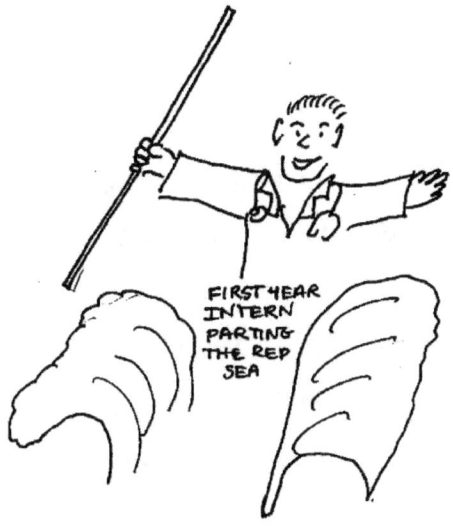

FIRST YEAR INTERN PARTING THE RED SEA

MD: Patients will sue you if you mess up (or if someone else messes up, and you ever treated the patient).

ND: Patients will thank you if you actually get them well.

Malpractice claims are down, but many doctors continue to practice "defensive medicine" in the illogical hope that they will beat the statistics and avoid the inevitable

lawsuits that all doctors deal with in their
lifetimes.

> **MD**: Patients do not want lifestyle change.
> **ND**: Patients do not want drugs.

In Washington state, despite insurance
equity between N.D.s and M.D.s, only 1-2%
of patients opt for lifestyle over drugs.

> **MD**: Patients do not pay you-insurance does.
> **ND**: Patients pay you-insurance doesn't.

Be aware that insurance tries to not pay you.
They delay or deny payments as a matter of
course because roughly a third of claims will
be dropped. Most M.D. office staff is
engaged full-time in the battle to get paid.

> **MD**: Your time is controlled by your job.
> **ND**: Your time is your own.

M.D. Or N.D.

If you like three week vacations, there really is only one career choice. If you like a full benefits package with retirement, then you need to choose the other.

    MD: You get a salary.
    ND: You are on your own.

While more Naturopathic Doctors are working on salary, it is still largely an entrepreneurial field. If you lack any other means to support yourself, becoming an N.D. is both terrifying and hunger inducing. Do not expect to beat the five-years-to-full-practice statistic for both fields.

    MD: You are on call. (Every other night, for life unless you choose a research-style position.)
    ND: You are on call only if you choose it. (Midwifery or terminal care.)

Being on call is a fascinating example of why more and more people are shying away from becoming M.D.s. A specialist may be the only one of his or her kind in a small city. They may be up all night several days in a row. Residents are limited to 24 hours at a time, but I guess specialists are made of sterner stuff?

MD: In five years, you will want to retire because the workload keeps getting heavier.

ND: In five years, you will finally be making enough money to live.

If you want to have the best primary care doctor, switch to someone six months into their practice. They make a great salary, and are yet to be busy. At five years, they are ten times busier and making the same amount, which is a burnout recipe. Meanwhile, the ND has been starving until

her referral base fills up and she is paid
more.

MD: You need 50k in equipment and support
staff to function as a doctor. (Not counting the
hospital needs.)

ND: You need a kitchen cabinet of herbs, your
head and your hands. (But are also often limited to
those.)

Fifty thousand is a very conservative
amount for a starting M.D. practice. Best to
plan for a business loan of five hundred
thousand to pay for office staff, equipment,
and malpractice insurance while waiting to
fill up.

I've always thought if everything hits the
fan it won't be conventional medicine that
continues to function. The system is based
on disposable everything, and diagnosis is
dependent on a network of laboratories

and machinery. If you're a pessimist, becoming an N.D. is a given.

MD: Prestige, power, and political influence.

ND: On the fringe, humility, patients as your boss and support.

Expect "What's that?" every time you say that you are a "Naturopathic Doctor." An M.D. knows that every single person in the room knows what they do and admires them for it.

There is no right choice. There is only a choice. I chose what I did because when I sat in silence it was what I was going to do anyway, and I realized that I didn't want to fight with my conventional colleagues or my nurses so I could spend as much time as I wanted with my patients.

It isn't about money, and it isn't about politics, it is about what you will love to do each day. If what you love is the adrenaline rush of saving people, you cannot find that as an N.D. If you love surgery, we're pretty small potatoes. If you already trust your gut and can make snap decisions, great. But if you don't feel satisfied until you've gotten to the root of the problem and love to spend lots of time with people, you'll never be happy in a standard medical model.

After reading about the differences, which career appeals to you more? Think about positions you've liked in the past and what you liked about them. Imagine yourself in each situation. Go back through the differences and circle which one is closest to you. Write down why.

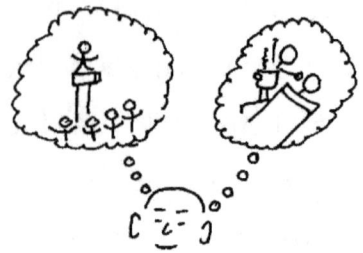

Some M.D.s still consider nutrition to be "unproven" as a treatment. They tell patients to go off berries while on chemo, but fast food is fine?

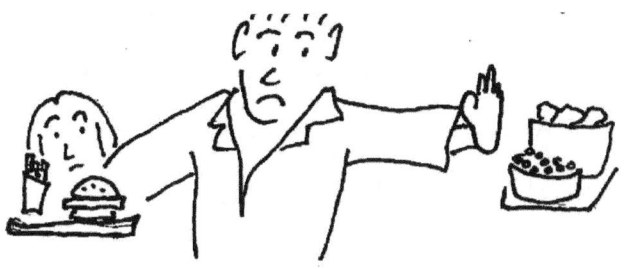

CHAPTER FOUR: HINDSIGHT IS 20/20

Despite flapping like a fish in the Sahara for years about this decision, I really had no choice of careers. When I was making my decision about whether to attend regular medical school or naturopathic medical school, I was only vaguely aware of my deep seated dislike of medicine and my strong preference for getting better on my own.

Here is an alphabet soup of reasons why I really had to be an N.D. If these look familiar, you may not need to go any farther. The decision was already made by genetics and nurture.

A) I was born on the west coast to parents who met in a commune. Already it was fated I'd go N.D., but read on.

B) My mother was the first person in her county to have a **home birth** in the last twenty years. I was that baby, and I made the news as an "alternative medicine" success before I could walk.

C) **My grandfather, currently 100 years old, was a chiropractor** and retired at 96. He sees me as his heir. (Update: Granpa died at 101. He'd fallen and they didn't think he'd be able to walk again. So he turned his face to the wall and went promptly.)

D) **I got sick getting vaccinated** four different times because my parents lost my shot records.

I still remember being dizzy and staggering against the wall after my fourth polio shot. The whole hospital hallway swung back and forth like a ship at sea. My mother disputes this story.

E) **An N.D. saved a dear relative's life** when grief twisted up her bowel and nothing else could be done.

He gave her several herbal laxatives and homeo-pathics for grief. Her M.D.s were considering a complete bowel removal to save her life. Later I studied under this N.D. I remember he had a BMW...from 1962.

F) **I went to N.D.s** throughout my childhood, even though I didn't know what they were. An N.D. screwed up a biopsy on my back, and pretty much put me off surgery as a career.

I avoided working with this N.D. later. He removed the stitches after only three days and they tore out. Sometimes we all need to know our limitations.

G) I was raised in a variety of religious traditions, which included a familiarity with Catholic, Buddhist, Protestant, Evangelical Christian, and Shamanistic traditions.

Spirituality is a part of most conversations in my practice. It isn't in most hospital wards.

H) When I broke my arm, I went to the only Osteopathic Hospital in the area. (It was closest, honest!)

I) In high school I had a mildly positive TB skin test. Rather than get the chest x-rays, which I knew were bad for me, I took a year of INH. I never received any oversight or follow up for this liver toxic drug. In retrospect, I am fortunate my liver was healthy, but the protocol was ridiculous. Public Health initiatives are sometimes better looking on paper than in actual practice.

J) **I always loved giving massages**, and was good at it well before I took classes.

I remember giving a course on massage in college and having one of my massages raffled off as a fundraiser.

K) With the exception of a few years of bingeing on penny candies, **I've always eaten healthy food**. My family has a lactose intolerance that makes us swell up if we have dairy.

It took me decades to admit how much dairy affects me. I'm still a recovering "dairyholic."

Christopher Maloney, N.D.

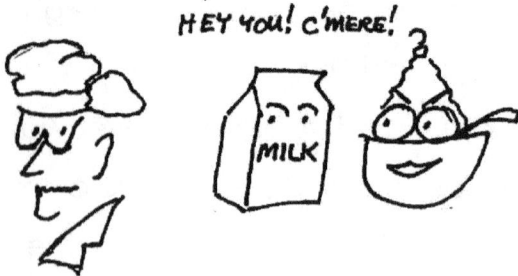

L) In Junior High **I created my own exercise routine** and followed it without oversight.

I would run for miles in bad shoes. In the process I learned discipline, what sore muscles feel like, and how good it is to be able to outrun your older brother.

M) I've always thought one of the holiest places in the world is a tall stand of conifers.

Nature is healing to me. Juxtapose that to how I feel about hospitals, and again it's obvious where I should be.

N) I went to a **liberal arts college** and majored in the theater arts. It was even spelled "theatre."

My march to a different drummer would have crashed and burned on the barricades of medical convention. Think Patch Adams without the humor.

O) **I love exotic food.** Thai or Indian food is preferable to standard American fare.

The reality is that I would have had nothing I liked to eat in most hospitals, which can be an issue if you're stuck in a place for twenty-four hours.

P) I love puzzles, the more complex, the better. **I don't like to have help or to have other people looking over my shoulder** while I solve it.

While patients benefit from this fascination, it isn't time efficient.

Conventional medicine rewards efficiency over solutions.

Q) In college, I got sick for six months. M.D.s weren't able to help me, and **I got better by myself**.

I would literally cough so hard I'd fall to the ground and try not to pass out. Anything could trigger it: laughter, cold air, even breathing hard. An M.D. told me I had bronchitis and to "just live with it." So I did breathing exercises for six months and gradually got better.

R) In graduate school, I volunteered to be medical students' first patient. During the interview, **I was far more comfortable than they were talking about the body**.
Interacting with me felt like it was a burden for them, while I was really excited to be there.

S) In graduate school, my hand went numb. The specialist told me to live with it because his hand was number. **I got better on my own.**

I had at least banged my hand on something. The hand expert had worn his watch too tight for months until he gave himself permanent nerve damage. Yes, he was Ivy League trained.

T) When we were overseas, **I preferred to sweat out a three-day fever** than to go to an overseas doctor.

U) **I went on intensive care wards with a friend and hated it.** They had to poke someone in the eye with a Q tip to get any response. I didn't want to work there.

The only patient I saw leave the ward alive was the one they didn't like. He had cancer and at one point just pulled out his IV drip and walked out. Everyone else died.

V) **I was mistaken for a doctor on the wards** and was asked to sign orders. I was also asked to do research for an infectious disease specialist on a rare disease we were discussing.

W) When I was doing my premedical studies, the students on either side of me were so ill they had to drop out. Out of three-hundred and fifty, **I was one of forty-five who made it through**. The rest only studied, I also worked full-time. I could do the grind, but it cost me gray hair.

X) **A medical friend ended up on amphetamines to make it through residency**. I got to watch him shake.

He was no ordinary person, with a rock solid faith in himself and the zeal to match. Nothing could have been less like him than for him to resort to self-prescribed meds.

Y) **My friends** in the Admissions/Financial Aid Office were silent about a regular medical career. But they all **were very enthusiastic about alternative medicine**. These were all professionals at finding good "fits" for students.

Z) I visited the N.D. school when it was closed. A janitor let me in, and the admissions officer happened to be there. I talked to the admission officer for two hours, applied and was admitted soon after for the following year. **In a world where many things are difficult, it seemed as if the way had been cleared for me**.

Christopher Maloney, N.D.

What would be an opposite life? I have a dear friend who was raised within the service model of conventional medicine. His entire extended family are M.D.s. His highest aspiration is to be like his father, who always places the patients first. I have never seen anyone so gleeful to work extra hours in the hospital. He receives endless energy from the process of meeting patients and staff. The happiest I have seen him is after a successful surgical intervention. Even if he told me tomorrow he was considering becoming an N.D., I would strongly try to dissuade him. No one I know is better suited or invested in the conventional M.D. route.

The blogosphere allows people to vent. Violent crime is dropping because the insult-o-sphere is here!

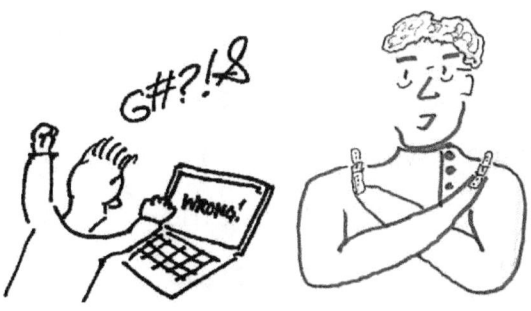

CHAPTER FIVE: PLACEBO VS. EVIDENCE

Is Naturopathic Medicine all a placebo effect? I would say that the reality of being a Naturopathic Doctor is dealing specifically with this issue on a very basic level. You can ignore it, get angry about it, or get over it, but you should deal with it because if you don't it will distract from your practice.

The majority of people you see will have an opinion about you. Those that see me overwhelmingly have been referred by multiple friends. They believe in their friends, not me. But if I manage to win their trust they have a whole framework of support to continue the lifestyle changes I prescribe.

When I get an outside referral, I tell them to read my website, which tells them an enormous amount about me. Again, patients with questions about whether or not I can help them usually self-select at that point not to see me.

But I am well aware that people who choose not to see me have questions about my practice. Let's deal with the most aggressive group in this area, the self-styled "skeptics."

Let me clarify if you're a N.D. those who call you names won't "believe" any evidence to the contrary. I've emailed all the major players in the skeptic crowd, and the replies I've received can be summed up by one old-time skeptic: "your evidence proves nothing." He didn't read it and even if he had it would not have changed anything. After dedicating forty years of his life to railing against anything alternative there really wasn't any room for him to alter his stance. He was invested in the status quo.

Before you waste years battling the skeptics, let me say that I've spent years debating them and providing them with medline (the clearinghouse for all peer-reviewed medical data) studies that they respond to with derision and no opposing data.

Before reading a "senior" skeptics' writings (there are less than ten cited regularly by others), always take a moment to peruse their own scientific contributions on medline. A reigning medline critic of Naturopathic Medicine published one scientific paper in 1976, and has done no human studies himself. Another has a tenured position at a leading medical institution, but has done only three tiny human studies within his field. How he is able to maintain tenure while not publishing, I do not know. Perhaps the most well-known online skeptic was never a researcher, and does not differentiate between his dislike of N.D.s and his dislike of postmodern thought.[iv]

The only major skeptic with the credentials to back up his criticisms mentions that the criteria he uses to "debunk" the effectiveness of alternative medicine would be too stringent for conventional medicine to pass scrutiny. He specifically takes issue with two standard deviations, P=0.05, being not significant enough to prove a treatment benefit. It is the standard for all drug and surgical trials. If it isn't significant, then we'd all better start from scratch.

When I began my journey on this career I was convinced that I would be the one to bring evidence-based medicine to those woo-woo Naturopaths. In retrospect the vast majority of diet and lifestyle changes that most N.D.s advocate are pretty well established. Many other groups are pushing for the same improvements in the Standard American Diet. Many of the herbs have decent small studies and great long-term safety profiles. A smaller number of herbs are well established as first line therapies for different illnesses. Think of peppermint for IBS. We recently added a clearinghouse for research relating directly to Naturopathic Medicine.[v] It simply isn't true that the research isn't being done, only that the critics don't believe the results.

The process of spending more time with the patient and fully answering their questions about their illness is a time honored technique that is encouraged in all medical practices. As some skeptics claim, much of what N.D.s do could be done by conven-tional practitioners, but the reality is that rarely do conventional practitioners have sufficient time.

Although much of Naturopathic Medicine has at least some evidence, critics take aim at the profession as a whole. The focus centers around three ideas:

1) you are killing patients by using unproven interventions,
2) you are killing patients by incompetently delaying "real" medical care, and/or
3) you are getting rich off gullible patients.

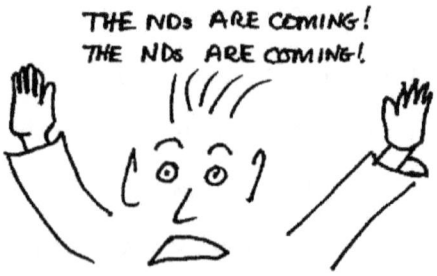

The evidence for the first assumption about N.D.s killing patients is lacking. None of the "great" skeptics can point to a major study that shows Naturopathic Doctors are killing anyone. Instead, they point to accumulated anecdotal reports of patient deaths where an alternative practitioner of any kind is mentioned. Then they lump N.D.s in with anyone who isn't an M.D. and claim causation where none has been proven or even hinted at in the original reports.

The medical evidence is clearly to the contrary. Case reports of side effects from supplements rarely implicate a licensed practitioner. It is almost entirely self-prescribing that goes awry, and the vast majority of patients seem to survive their experimentation with alternative medicine even with a complete lack of oversight.

Christopher Maloney, N.D.

Every time a celebrity illness or worsening of symptoms can be blamed on alternative medicine the critics will leap on it. In recent years Apple founder Steve Job's death was blamed on his use of alternative medicine.

A quick fact check would show that Jobs had pancreatic cancer with a six to eighteen month window of life. He had a surgical removal of the tumor in 2008 and can be seen telling a graduating class at Stanford that he is cancer free. When the cancer returned, of course he pursued alternatives, because there were no conventional options left. But it would be wrong to say that alternatives did anything to shorten his life. Far from killing him, alternatives may have provided him with some pain relief during his last days. He sought conventional treatments first despite their lack of effect and delayed any alternative treatments until it was too late to do anything but help him with pain.

The second issue is that N.D.s are somehow preventing patients from getting real help from conventional doctors. If N.D.s are in fact delaying "real" medical care, the malpractice lawyers have not discovered it. M.D.s are sued for negligence, while N.D.s seem somehow "immune."

The malpractice insurance industry does not seem to be concerned with any delays. N.D. malpractice insurance remains miniscule compared to M.D. insurance rates, so the insurance industry is not concerned about it. In states where N.D.s receive insurance reimbursement equality with M.D.s we still don't see an increase in legal involvement. So the only people concerned with the delay of conventional care are the skeptics.

Christopher Maloney, N.D.

From my own practical experience, patients maintain a variety of doctors simultaneously. Most turn to me only when conventional treatments have been unsuccessful, and I encourage them to maintain their existing doctor as well. A team approach gives the best care.

The underlying assumption about delay by the skeptics is that N.D.s have nothing to bring to the table. To test this idea naturopathic care has been added to a conventional hospital model. In the German hospital in Blankenstein, long-term follow up showed significant benefit from Naturopathic treatment in addition to conventional treatment. Individualized patient care by N.D.s gave greater relief than conventional treatment alone.[vi]

The third point, that N.D.s are in their professions to get rich, doesn't bear out with the salaries. N.D.s make less than primary care doctors, and far, far less than specialists. Since N.D. schools require the same premedical requirements, one would assume only martyrs would go to N.D. school when they could go to M.D. school and make at least twice as much.[vii]

But the three points of criticism have little or no meaning for the majority of patients an N.D. sees. Most of my patients have already been to their conventional doctors and did not like their options. Many are already self-prescribing all sorts of things (which they haven't told their conventional doctors). I've seen everything self-prescribed, from drinking soap or urine to a range of starvation exercises or caustic purgatives.

My job is to walk a patient through what is known about the illness and how whatever they are doing is likely to affect that situation. Rarely am I able to dissuade patients from doing anything that seems the least bit effective to them, but often I am able to move them onto something less toxic. I would say that I'm far more conservative than the bulk of my patients about what I'd prescribe and how fast I expect it to be effective. Those conventional doctors who work with me refer to me because they know I'm able to move patients away from damaging alternative treatments and still give them options.

For those determined to find the evidence itself, have a look at my website www.maloneymedical.com under What Do I Treat or have a look at some of the diseases I discuss on my blog Alternative Health Answers. If you are reading medline, get to know the individuals writing the

Cochrane reviews. Even on the meta-analysis level, the assumptions of the authors profoundly affect the outcome. I am encouraged that ten years ago a search for alternative medicine turned up a hundred thousand hits on medline. Now the number is closer to two hundred thousand. Keep in mind that the vast majority of what I find on medline has not been indexed to alternative medicine because it has only been catalogued to a specific herb. The system wasn't set up for the complexities of an N.D.'s practice.

Christopher Maloney, N.D.

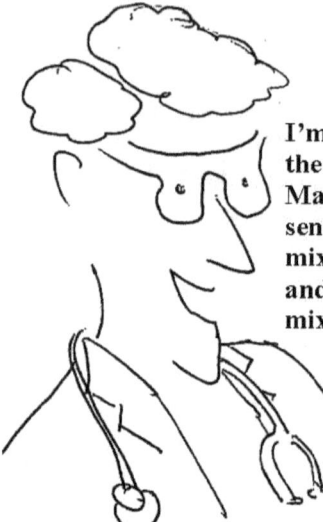

I'm constantly amazed by the number of supplements. Many of them make no sense. I've seen probiotics mixed with antibiotic herbs, and constipating agents mixed with laxatives!

CHAPTER SIX: SUPPLEMENT SALESMEN OR WORSE?

I think the average person wants to feel that a doctor will find out what is wrong with them and make them feel better without hurting them or making them bankrupt. For the average person, a bad doctor encompasses several things: a snake oil salesman, or a fanatic, or an incompetent.

Beyond the simple evidence debate is the morality of being in alternative medicine. As a profession on the fringe, N.D.s have to deal with legitimate concerns about the nature of their practice and their ethics. Within alternative medicine are many people who could be described as supplement salesmen, snake oil hawkers, fanatics, or incompetents. It is unfortunate that such people exist, but here I'd like to discuss how I've addressed each of these possible criticisms.

SUPPLEMENT SALESMEN

One of the criticisms I hear about my profession is that most of us sell the products we prescribe. It limits patient choice and pressures patients more than if they were simply allowed to shop elsewhere.

It is true that many N.D.s sell supplements in their offices but it is also true that quality control for the supplement industry is highly variable. It is also true that the vast majority of supplements sold can be refilled online from warehouse sites at costs less than N.D.s can purchase wholesale and without requiring another prescription. So not only are N.D.s making less money, they also have no prescription monopoly on resupplying their patients.

N.D.s have not learned how, like optometrists, to get their prescriptions to expire within a year and force patients to return.

SNAKE OIL

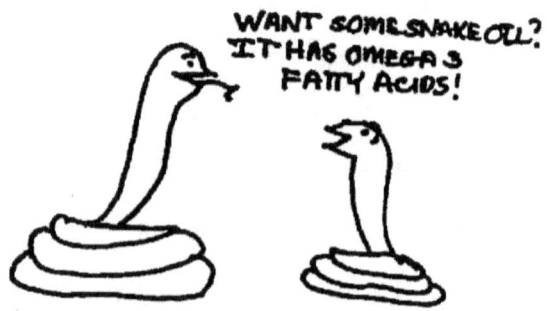

So, am I a snake oil salesman? I do prescribe supplements, for which I provide peer-reviewed, evidence-based medline research. I have struggled with promoting specific supplements because I do not like the conflict of interest it generates, but many of my patients were not getting what I prescribed otherwise. Alternative medicine pharmacies are not available, and I need to be certain that what I prescribe actually has an active herb or the proper amount of amino acid that we need to match the clinical results in the research.

My understanding of snake oil is that it doesn't have any medical research behind it, that it is unique to the salesperson and not available anywhere else, and that it was seriously overpriced. Everything I prescribe has research that I provide to the patient, it is available from multiple sources, and I have been known to arrange for patients to purchase at wholesale prices when the supplement gets too expensive. So I am not a snake oil salesman.

But are there snake oil salesmen within alternative medicine? Absolutely. Any time an individual patents a medicine, they are not doing so for the benefit of the patient. Every week I see miracle cures that have been priced out of the range that a normal person could afford them. But it is the individual with the degree, not the degree itself, that has decided to put profit above patient care. Patients sense this, regardless of the profession, and will say it simply as: "he's all about the money."

FANATIC

Am I a fanatic? Many of my patients use me for confession of their health and lifestyle "crimes." They list off all the sugary treats they love, and wait for me to take them all away.

I don't, because I am primarily interested in compliance: the ability of a patient to follow the treatment plan. Other patients come in to me convinced that I am a raw food, vegan, yoga zen guru. They are shocked that I still have my mercury fillings or that I eat everything. But because I am far from perfect, I can meet each patient where they are, without judgment. My only goal is each person's increased health, whether that be on Atkins or as a vegan, on multiple drugs or drug free. It is what will work for that person in the long run, not some fad or crash program. So I am not a fanatic.

Are there fanatics within Naturopathic Medicine? Oh my, yes! So many of my colleagues have their sacred cows (or sacred tofu burgers). It is our equivalent of specialties. One person might think that environmental toxins are the cause of all ills (they probably don't help your ills, but I'm not convinced they are the cause of all problems). Another might think that every person needs a thousand dollars in supplements just to function. A third might put everyone on the same diet, because it's "how we all should eat." We all think our way is best, which is why any wise patient will shop around. Chances are good that you can eventually find an N.D. that agrees that at least part of your life is healthy. I remember one N.D. promoting eating at Burger King.

To be fair, my sacred cow is research. I work very hard to admit that a therapy might have some benefit when it hasn't been researched. Not every-thing needs a journal write-up to be valuable. But since I am willing to consider anything that might help the patient, I keep my research bias under control.

INCOMPETENCE

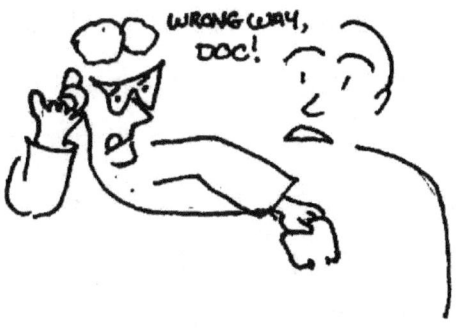

Am I incompetent? This is an issue I wrestle with, because I am a generalist in a specialist world. If all your podiatric rheumatologist treats is your big toe, how can I expect to match his knowledge in that area? Fortunately, he and his colleagues continually research the best treatments for the big toe, so in many cases I can benefit from the knowledge of multiple experts and pass that information on to you.

I will not see a patient that I feel I cannot help, and I have put into place a money back guarantee to be sure that the patients feel they are getting value from our visits. I can say that in areas I lack knowledge I immediately seek it, and I will educate myself about any therapy, no matter how far fetched or how invasive. I have only had patients leave when they are well or when they found another program that I did not offer. And many chronic patients return to me because after going the rounds of the specialists they find my approach to be the most helpful.   When I question patients about how they've done without me after several year, they tell me that when they were doing the program that we set out, they got better.   But then they forgot or had other priorities and stopped doing the things that helped and they got worse. So I would judge myself as competent, with constant improvement possible.

Are there incompetents within Naturopathic medicine? Yes and no. There are people who add little but a listening ear, but that is not without its merits. Because of the amounts of time N.D.s spend with their patients and the relatively common practice of having both a PCP and an N.D. work on a case, true incompetence is rarely felt by the patient from even the least well-informed N.D.

NEGLIGENCE VS COMPETENCE

The legal standard of incompetence seems to be severely injuring a patient, which is extremely rare among the N.D. circles.

I don't respect the lowering of standards to this level, and I wish we held our medical professionals to the same levels of other professions. Shouldn't a specialist that is not able to provide any relief to your condition wave you out the door without charge? We expect this of our plumbers, our carpenters, and our mechanics. Our restaurants, our supermarkets, and retail stores provide some assurance that satisfaction will be provided.

In modern medicine, we are now assured that our confidentiality will be kept, implying that previously it was not. But when was the last time you saw a hospital advertising: "satisfaction guaranteed or your money back?" Wouldn't it be far less expensive than waiting for highly dissatisfied consumers to sue for malpractice?

But doctors must charge like lawyers, for time. And if you think about the six minutes you get with a specialist for your several hundred dollars, then the cost of healthcare far exceeds any other commodity. I do not have all the answers for the healthcare crisis, but I am part of the solution: an individual doctor taking responsibility for providing excellent care.

Christopher Maloney, N.D.

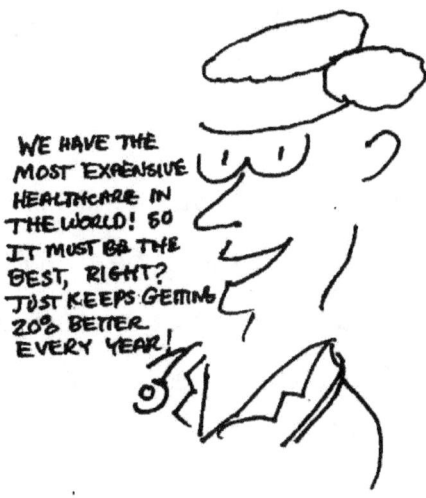

CHAPTER SEVEN: A BANKRUPTING
MACHINE?

Please recall: the average person wants to feel that a doctor will find out what is wrong with them and make them feel better without hurting them or making them bankrupt.

A basic well-established fact: **62% of personal bankruptcies in the United States are caused by medical expenses** (Warren

67

report, 2009). **Three-fourths of those had health insurance but were still bankrupted by copayments** over an extended chronic illness.[viii]

The financial ruin rate would be somewhat acceptable if the medical care were necessary, evidence based, and curative. Those are criteria that are surprisingly difficult to meet.

I recommend <u>Money Driven Medicine</u> by Maggie Mahar for those who believe that modern medicine is driven by science. The author does a truly chilling job of showing that modern medicine is in very serious trouble. (I have no connection to the book, and receive nothing for endorsing it).

Myth 1: We Only Receive Necessary Treatment

Among the most serious myths is that idea that modern medical practice is dictated by science and that evidence based medicine is the standard. In reality, the amount of care a patient receives is largely due to the number of doctors available. Each doctor may do his or her job completely competently, but the combination of treatments and drugs is often not coordinated or overseen.

Those who receive more care actually have less quality of care given and tend to die sooner. Dartmouth has done a wonderful job of documenting this year after year. Here is a brief excerpt:

"during the first six months following hip fracture, patients using academic medical centers in high-spending areas had 82% more physician visits, 26% more imaging exams, 90% more diagnostic tests, and 46% more minor surgery. Nevertheless, patients in high-intensity regions had higher mortality rates and worse quality scores.[ix]"

Myth 2: At Least I Have A Diagnosis

The second myth that patients experience is that all of the technology they are subjected to will give them an accurate diagnosis of their illness. Most patients are aware that the treatments for their illness, if any exist, have side effects. But we are assured that at least the diagnosis will be accurate. But autopsies tell a different story:

"One hundred eleven malignant neoplasms in 100 patients had been either undiagnosed or misdiagnosed, and in 57 patients, the immediate cause of death could be attributed to the malignant neoplasm. The discordance between clinical and autopsy diagnoses of malignant neoplasms in this study is 44%, which is similar to previously reported studies.[x]"

An analysis of autopsy reports found: "Twenty-six autopsy series reported both major and class I error rates. The median error rate was 23.5% (range, 4.1%-49.8%) for major errors (a major error means doctors missed diagnosing a disease that directly contributed to death) and 9.0% (range, 0%-20.7%) for class I errors (a class I error means doctors missed the disease that caused death) .[xi]"

If we paraphrase the information, we find that doctors vary widely in how they treat and vary widely in how accurately they can predict the correct disease and even the cause of death.

Myth 3: We Have the Finest Healthcare.

Health care in the U.S. costs twice as much as what is spent in Japan, which has a higher life expectancy and a lower infant mortality rate.[xii]

Myth 4: We do not ration care. They do.

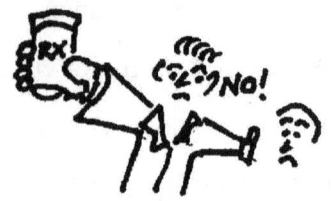

John Hopkins found that for that the top fifteen procedures that are rationed in other countries account for just 3% of U.S. health care spending, not enough to make a major difference. P.XVI

We also do not have as many hospital beds as in rationing countries.[xiii]

Myth 5: It's all due to malpractice insurance.

We do file 50% more malpractice claims than in the UK or Australia and 350% more than Canada, but awards for U.S. citizens are lower than those given in the UK or Canada. Malpractice payments have been growing at 5% a year in the U.S. while in the UK and Canada they have been growing from 10-28%.   Overall, malpractice payments represent less than 1% of health care spending.[xiv]

Karen Davis of the Commonwealth Fund says why we pay more for health care in the U.S.: we pay higher prices for the same services, we have higher administrative costs, and we perform more complex, specialized procedures. She also notes a wide disparity in both services and outcomes, crediting the fee-for-service model for maintaining a lack of standardization within U.S. healthcare. (Commonwealth President's address, 2005).

Myth 6: It was better in the good old days.

Christopher Maloney, N.D.

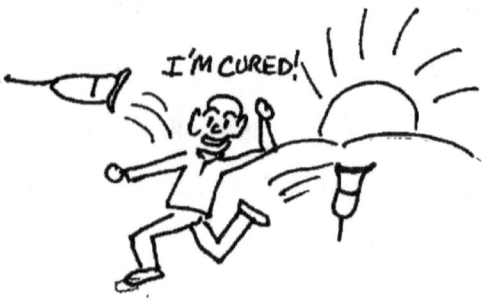

A very brief history of conventional medicine in the United States:

Up until the 1930s patients paid out-of-pocket for services. (As they continue to do for N.D.s) The poor went to the hospitals.

In 1929, people could not pay for the hospitals at all. Blue Shield was created as hospital insurance simply to keep the hospitals from closing. It funded hospitals based on their costs, so they had no incentive to cut and every incentive to increase costs. The AMA set up Blue Cross because it agreed to pay the M.D. whatever he asked and headed off any move toward a mandatory, government-run insurance program.

During World War II, wage controls made it possible to increase wages only by adding benefits. Hospital plans went from seven million to twenty six million subscribers. By 1954, sixty percent of the population had some type of hospital insurance, fifty percent had surgical insurance and twenty-five percent had medical insurance, but only for in-hospital services. Employer-based health care meant that only the healthy could have health care. The old and sick could not hold down the jobs necessary to apply.

By 1965 seventy percent of the country had hospital insurance, but more than half of seniors had no insurance. In 1962, President Kennedy had pushed for medicare, but the AMA opposed medicare and it was defeated. President Johnson compromised by allowing hospitals and doctors to set whatever price they "needed" to charge. By the time it passed in 1965, the bill covered seniors for hospitals and doctors. It also included poor families. By 1970, the amount paid out by taxpayers had tripled. In the years from 1960 to 1970, the overall health bill rose from $27 billion to $73 billion.[xv]

President Nixon passed the first HMO act and set up a national health insurance plan. But his impeachment derailed the process. By 1980, health care spending was up to $257 billion. Medicare and Medicaid had grown by 600 percent. President Reagan stopped the blank checks in 1983 by dividing up payments based on procedures.

The market was given its sway, and for a time HMOs became the most hated non-caregivers as they attempted to ration care.

In 1990 the nation spent $700 billion on care. In 2000 the HMOs capitulated and the cost of family coverage rose 73% from 2000-2005 as they passed on increased costs to the consumer. By 2006, the nation spent three times what it had in 1990.[xvi]

Myth 7: We Have Safeguards On the System

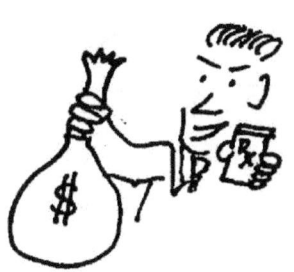

Here, take this. Now, you decide, is my drug safe?

For-profit hospitals are beholden to their stockholders. Not-for profit hospitals are beholden to their bond issuers. Both need to be in the black and make a decent profit.

The FDA is monitoring our drug supply. **Drug companies provide more than half the FDA's financial support through user fees**.

79% of the drug unit time is spent on new drug reviews.[xvii]

The drug makers spent $19 billion on research and $45 billion for advertising, while pocketing $31 billion in profits. (Families USA, 2002)

Myth 8: We Can Pay For It.

Half of U.S. workers have less than $25k in savings. Two thirds have less than $50k. The average person in 40-50s is $20k in debt (not including mortgages). One in ten workers and one in five retirees has more than $250k.[xviii]

My apologies if the above seems harsh, but it does not reflect on brilliant and ethical individual M.D.s within the system. The system as a whole has never functioned in a cost-effective, sustainable manner.

The inability of the system to maintain itself does not mean you cannot have a brilliant career as an M.D. But it factors in greatly to the dissatisfaction that current M.D.s have with their careers. The natural expansion of this dissatisfaction is "boutique medicine," a process in which the M.D. contracts directly with the patient for care. If you look back, this is a return to the pre-hospital model of care, and may provide greater satisfaction for some M.D.s. Others have come to terms with the idea of being salaried employees and are finding ways to maintain a sane lifestyle within the framework of the current system. A dear friend of mine has managed to carve out four weeks of vacation for himself every year, but does not directly see patients as a result. So it is possible to have a good life within the current system despite its shortcomings.

A number of my patients cannot be helped by conventional medicine. They need an operation only they can do: a spouse-ectomy!

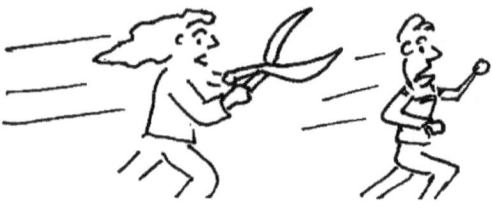

CHAPTER EIGHT: QUESTIONS AND ANSWERS

Some of the following are of broad interest, but several are more specific.

"I wonder why Naturopathic medicine has not made its mark in mainstream America?"

Given that there are probably 5,000 licensed NDs in the U.S., up from 2,000 ten years ago, I think we're doing pretty well. For comparison, there are at least 50,000 active Chiropractors and 70,000 acupuncturists. They pale compared to 500,000 active practicing MDs.

In states where we have schools, we've achieved primary care status, insurance reimbursement, and we all can get malpractice insurance.

There was a landmark case that we lost in the late 1970's that failed to get us national stature. Alternative medicine as a whole received a huge boost in 1989 when the AMA lost an anti-trust suit in the Supreme Court brought by the chiropractic associations.[xix] Up until that point an MD could have his license revoked for associating with an alternative doctor. So the answer is that we've been here in tiny numbers but are finally rapidly growing since the environment has opened up somewhat.

I say somewhat because Anthem here in Maine still maintains an exclusion at the back of their handbook for patients looking for naturopathic care. Although I have primary care status in Maine, all my services are specifically not covered, including those services that are covered for MDs or DOs. There is no legitimate medical reason for a blanket exclusion, but the Maine Medical Association has actively opposed any coverage for us and some of their members advise Anthem Blue Cross Blue Shield about coverage. No coverage means the hospitals aren't willing to have us practice onsite and limits our patient base to those who can afford it.

"Are you supporting yourself, and how long will it take for me to be able to support myself?"

As with any medical practice, it takes five years to get full. In my case, I work half-time to pay the bills while caring for my children half-time. My wife was able to leave her state job and pursue her own interests because I'm able to support us working half-time. I've also failed previously, and succeeded mildly. (I'm writing a second book: How to Fail and Succeed in Alternative Medicine, about how to make it.)

Do Naturopathic Schools teach evidence-based medicine? What about things like homeopathy? Do you believe in it?

The search for evidence is lifelong. Much of what you will be taught in Naturopathic Medical school is based on tradition, and at times based on the professor's personal ideology.

One area I was particularly disgusted with was homeopathy. In a confrontation with a "homeo-head" I was dared to consume a bottle of homeopathics to prove my point. I did so, and the resulting four-day headache defied all my attempts at resolution. In desperation, I asked for help.

Resolution came after taking a single pellet and immediately spitting it out. To this day I do not believe in homeopathics, but I can say the correct combinations have solved my children's illnesses with a rapidity that continues to astound me (when I use the wrong combinations, nothing happens. Two years ago it took twenty-one attempts, but at the twenty-first try a three-month wheeze resolved in minutes).

I do have seventeen pages of medline data on homeopathy under <u>What Do I Treat</u> at www.maloneymedical.com. The meta-analyses are mixed, but we do have something like five thousand randomized controlled trials done.

A number of other areas of Naturopathic practice have negative support. Applied kinesiology is no better than chance. (Note: this refers to the closed supplement bottle approach. Older versions of the technique were practiced with a substance on the tongue, which can be as accurate as a allergy blood test), although it is experiencing a resurgence at my alma mater, NCNM, right now. Ear candling has no support, but will still be taught. And a number of herbs simply aren't doing what we think they should (Echinacea was never effective against colds in the oral form. The original German studies were based on injecting it, something we don't do. It does raise white blood cell counts, but I'm not convinced this is anything more than irritation and cross reaction by the immune system to the large polysaccharide molecules).

Christopher Maloney, N.D.

Take a moment with me and look at conventional medicine for comparison. Is the emperor wearing any clothes?

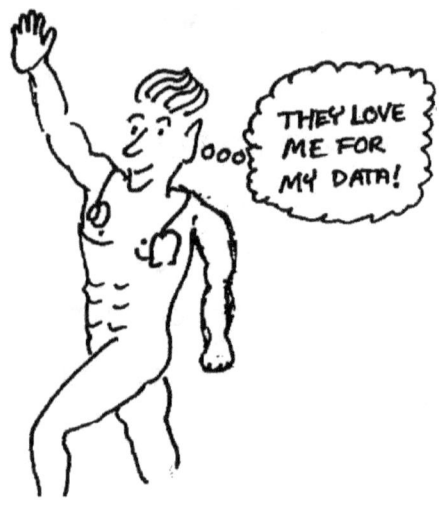

I just did twenty pages of research for a patient with deep vein thrombosis (blood clot). The presumed treatment is coumadin, a blood thinner, and the highest risk time is in the first five days. He was told to take two aspirin, not given coumadin, and had no office visits scheduled. His surgeon did not tell him about the blood clot risk although it is quite common. By the time he thought to call me (after days in agony) the clot had resolved. From my point of view, an extract of horse chestnut has shown some ability to lessen the pain and help resolve the clot. I wouldn't expect the conventional doctors to know my stuff, but they often don't know the best evidence-based treatments.

So, while I would agree that Naturopathic Medical education can be improvement and made more evidence-based, I think the same criticism can apply to conventional medical schools.

"MD's... look like they are offering everything that ND's can and more.

"I also heard about the Echinacea study...I fear that more studies such as this will come out and...send the profession into another a decline like it experienced 50 years ago."

Christopher Maloney, N.D.

(from a student in San Francisco)

I think the real question is whether Naturopathic medicine will be either absorbed or become irrelevant in the next few years. I think we'll eventually be absorbed into the mainstream conventional model, but I don't think we'll lose our distinctive profession. We've got a clinic out here that features a collaborative integrative practice. They wanted to hire me, but they wanted me to pay $800+ for a single day a month at their clinic. I asked to look at the books, and they were almost empty of patients, because Mainers have the lowest per-capita out-of-pocket health care spending in the country. The clinic continues to lose money. Every year they ask me for a donation, because they see themselves as the future of healthcare. I checked recently, and all the MDs have second, "real" jobs within the conventional system. I've seen this same problem with other integrative models.

The Cancer Treatment Centers of America have N.D.s on staff, but I have heard from patients that they are not referred to as doctors. I sent a patient there to receive a novel Interleukin 2 treatment I had recommended that had excellent results in the German studies, but they killed her with radiation instead. I was never contacted or consulted for follow up. Equality is not as common as it may appear in the integrative model. So N.D.s are not at a place where they will be absorbed anytime soon.

But can't the regular doctors just do what we do? Recently we had a D.O. who treats with alternative methods run out of the state because his board refused to renew his license. The boards out west may be more lenient, but boards tend to be more conservative than the average doctor.

Forgive me, but San Francisco is hardly representative of the country. If you just want to practice in the city, then it may be possible to be an M.D. and do what you want. But almost anywhere we're licensed you'll run into more legal issues as an M.D. practicing "on the edge" of your licensure. My board is made up of mostly N.D.s who do the same things I do.

If we look at the direction of N.D.s fifty years into the future, let's have a look at the D.O.s Are they alternative? Not anymore. Here's an update from their national board. I don't see much manipulation anymore, and most of them are looking to become M.D.s now.

"During recent decades, a movement away from osteopathic medicine's traditionally primary-care-focused and separate training/practice system has occurred. Nearly all osteopathic hospitals closed or were integrated into allopathic hospital systems, student clinical training expanded into venues with MD education programs, fewer DO graduates pursued traditional primary care training, 60% entered training programs of the Accreditation Council for Graduate Medical Education, and DO and MD specialty practice integration became widespread.[xx]"

Nothing wrong with joining up, but the whole point was to be a separate but equal group. But what happened to the D.O.s is likely to happen to the N.D.s When I was on the conventional medical track I was encouraged to apply to both M.D. and D.O. schools because "D.O. schools take a slightly lower grade point average." Nothing about the difference in medical philosophy, the uniqueness of osteopathic manipulation, or the family practice focus. So M.D. students getting into D.O. schools pushed the curriculum closer and closer to the M.D. model until there isn't much distinction.

Even if the schooling stayed separate, once you enter into the insurance reimbursement model the medicine you practice has to change. When I surveyed my graduating class, all of us wanted legal equality with the M.D.s but none of us wanted anything to do with insurance.

My Oregon classmates now take insurance, or insurance takes them. If you will be reimbursed for a set procedure, and not for another procedure, how much freedom do you have conventionally or alternatively?

But will the Naturopathic profession be shown to have no research behind it and fade away? We're going to continue to see negative reports about alternative medicine because it is a major competitor to the pharmaceutical industry. Negative press makes the news, but the overwhelming reality is that most of the reports are mixed or show some merit. The Echinacea study you mentioned does show it doesn't stop the flu when given to healthy college students, but it does raise the white blood count, which might help.

A few years back, there were more than one hundred thousand medline citations for complementary medicine. Now there are two hundred thousand. Keep in mind that this is not an actual listing, because medline wasn't set up for alternative medicine, and I usually need to do an herb/supplement/dietary specific subsearch to find any information.

Christopher Maloney, N.D.

Even the most conservative skeptic (E. Ernst) estimates that 7.4% of alternative medicine is evidence-based. For comparison, a Duke researcher estimated that 80% of conventional medical practice lacks randomized, controlled trials, including many of the common practices done in emergency rooms and surgical wards. I found a lovely site that actually lists the data on placebo vs. evidence-based medicine in various conventional medical fields showing a very wide range.[xxi]

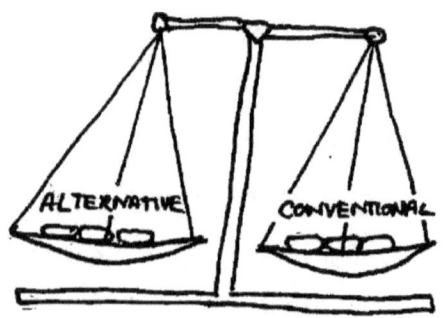

I'll just keep working away at my 7.4%, which I have to laugh at and say that in any general practice the studies say that stress is a factor in 80% of outpatient illness. Diet and lifestyle affect stress, and I work with diet and lifestyle. So I'm using evidence-based interventions on at least 80% of my patients.

As to a practice in San Francisco, ask any of your laid back M.D. colleagues if they could work twenty hours a week. In a cash-only practice. Without being on call. Without advertising. It's awesome. I cured (at least temporarily) an asthmatic in 2.5 hours today. Complete physical/emotional/spiritual work up. She stopped coughing when I treated her and she started dealing with the loss of her father when she was eight. There isn't anywhere else in the world I want to be right now.

Christopher Maloney, N.D.

I love that every year diet and fitness trends peak
in January. In Maine that's a recipe for frustration
and disaster with ice roads and snow closures.
We should move the New Year push to the first
day of spring!

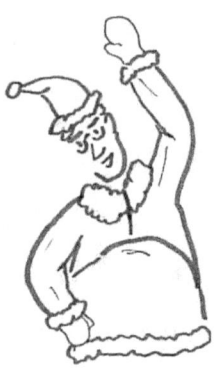

*"Why are plant based medicines better
than pharmaceuticals? Aren't pharmaceuticals more precisely engineered to
treat the problem and without all the
hundreds of other errant chemicals that
the plant based medicine will carry?"*

While we can quantify to some degree
the damage done by pharmaceuticals, it is
harder to figure out what is happening with

herbs. Let's start by saying that 98% of all herbs are taken by patients without oversight. They may inform their doctor, but only somewhere around 25% do so. So we can't say for certain what the extent of herb/drug interaction is.

We can, however, get a pretty good idea of mortality rates for herbs. Once an herb hits the public eye conventional doctors are very good at assigning blame to it. Ephedra was responsible for possibly six deaths before being pulled from the market. Kava kava was responsible for 34 liver failures, a number that turned out to be only 11 deaths that had been triple reported. In the extensive follow-up, only one of the 11 deaths did not have significant liver toxic drug intake as well. In the final analysis, the European commission resolved that no liver deaths could be attributed to kava kava. But it remains illegal in Europe and Canada.

Christopher Maloney, N.D.

(Update: Europe quietly resumed selling kava in 2008.)

Compare this to the recent Vioxx debacle. Several hundred thousand deaths possible. One of its closely tied drug brethren (Celebrex) continues to be marketed.

One hundred thousand deaths can be attributed to drug intake every year in the U.S. alone. This is drug intake within the regular prescription range, with proper oversight. Another hundred thousand patients are sickened to the point of needing hospitalization from the regular, standard dosing of drugs. We just don't see those numbers in alternative medicine.

But I remember thinking that if herbs could just be harnessed, broken down into their constituent parts, then we'd make some useful discoveries. That was one of my focuses in becoming an naturopathic doctor. Turns out I was wrong.

A subset of the current drugs is purified from the original plants. But a lot of the newer drugs are based on test tube processes that tend to go wrong in human testing. The older discoveries, things like antibiotics and aspirin, made us think we could improve on Mother Nature. We could tease out a metabolic process and make a drug that would just affect that process. But we failed to take into account the incredible complexity of the reactions that take place within the human body.

Take something as basic as ascorbic acid, vitamin C. We need vitamin C and it is water soluble. Turns out you can only absorb 250mg or so through your gut lining, and the rest becomes "expensive waste." Funny thing, the record for one of my patients is 88 grams of vitamin C. That's 88 grams consumed on a single day, without diarrhea or other ill effects. I still don't know where he put it all, and I certainly wouldn't prescribe that much. But I can consume 2-5 grams without the osmotic diarrhea that should result. Is it being consumed by my gut bacteria? Perhaps.

Of course, we all know the "best" way to get vitamin C is through a pill, which can give you the vitamin C of six oranges. Only about 16% of the vitamin C is absorbed that way, so in order to get your 250 mg you need to take a bit more (a gram and a half). On the other hand, if you eat an orange 96% of the orange's vitamin C will be absorbed directly.

I chose vitamin C because we've known about it for hundreds of years. It's a natural, essential nutrient, and has a very low toxicity. But we're still arguing about whether too much vitamin C could be harmful.

Take the vitamin C discussion and multiply it by a thousand for some synthetic compound that is supposed to mimic a body process. Will it be absorbed? What will happen to it in the body? Are there other body processes that will try and use that compound and cause unforeseen side effects? How will it be broken down by the body? What stages will it go through during that breakdown? Are any of those stages extremely toxic? In a patient with a slowed liver function, could those toxic byproducts build up and cause serious problems?

When you start asking those complicated questions, some curious answers come back about herbs. Take an herb like black cohash, which is used for menopause, and which may affect hot flashes by affecting estrogen levels in the body. First, it doesn't affect estrogen directly, it affects the hormones that generate estrogen. But doesn't that cause increased breast cancer risk? It might, but there are eight different compounds within black cohash that block the growth of breast cancer cells. So the whole herb might be a lot better for women than a synthetic extract of the "active" ingredient.

Another example. St. John's Wort was promoted as an antidepressant herb. A number of companies started promoting a standardized extract of the "active" ingredient, but they had to change it a couple times because they weren't sure of which was the active ingredient. Then a big study came out saying that St. John's Wort was no better than placebo for depression. They didn't say that the study was a three part study: St. John's Wort vs. Zoloft vs.

Placebo. The placebo group did better than either St. John's Wort or Zoloft. Neither showed any effect, but only St. John's Wort got the negative publicity. Later on, they did more studies and found that St. John's Wort is effective again. But the "active" ingredient may be that St. John's Wort speeds up the liver's ability to process drugs and other compounds. It is so good at speeding up the liver it inactivates birth control pills (Another negative media report). But that ability may help depressed people process out neuropeptide compounds that are contributing to their depression.

So I've come full circle from wanting to purify a new drug to recognizing the complexity of the system we're trying to heal. If you wanted to pigeon-hole me and ask me what I do, I'd say forget supplements long-term. The average patient will stop taking even the most effective supplements after two to three years anyway. I use supplements as an interim step to getting people on a better diet. Ninety percent of what I want people to use long-term you could use in a salad or as seasoning. It might not taste that good to you and I, but I work very hard to find something the patient enjoys and finds pleasant. It becomes part of their culinary world, not their drug or supplement world.

I can use bile salts in the short term to drop cholesterol, and continue to support a person's diet long-term rather than hook him on statins. I can use mushroom capsules to raise a white blood cell count, and turmeric to oppose the negative after-effects of chemotherapy. So of course my herbs don't have the same side effects as pharmaceuticals. Of course it is safer! It's just dried food. I take "do no harm" very seriously. Why would you use something like antibiotics to try and kill a mild virus when garlic can do it better? Seriously. Garlic is both antiviral and antifungal and will kill everything that amoxicillin will with the exception of the pneumonia bug.

The real problem with the drugs is that we have no data on the long-term effects of any of these drugs. No one is doing thirty-year trials. We have six-day, six-week and maybe six-month trials on drugs that we tell people to take forever. There is no data to support the long-term, chronic use of most of these compounds, and very good data that side effect pictures mount over time.

As a society we need to move toward food and away from the drugs. But the current legal situation is that if a doctor takes you off your drugs and something happens he or she will get sued. Even if you are having side effects, it is safer for your doctor to maintain your medication. It's a backwards world where synthetic compounds are safe and food is risky.

To an acupuncturist specifically looking to specialize in oncology in Maine.

Great plan! No, getting an additional Naturopathic Doctor degree won't help unless you're working with a specialty group.

Medical oncologists will most likely do one of the following: love you, accept referrals without referring back, disregard your medical opinion, treat you like a support staff, and/or ignore you entirely as a freak regardless of the number of degrees you have. Some of them will alternate. Patients will love you and will seek you out because of your focus.

By focusing on a single area, you will become an expert in that area but end up treating everything (cancer is not a single disease, it encompasses the spectrum).

On the other hand, if you want to run an alternative center, the secondary degree will be very helpful. You can also use the second degree as a springboard to work with Cancer Treatment Centers of America, who may still treat you like support staff.

If I were trying to specialize in oncology acupuncture, I'd spend my time in the hospitals while still studying as a student, working with patients to create functional protocols. Then I'd write my first book of protocols before I graduated and spend a couple of years traveling around New England working for others before settling in Maine. Then my pull area for my practice would be down to Boston and back.

So you're on the right track, but don't expect to make a living in Maine straight out. Come with a six month/year cushion

Christopher Maloney, N.D.

and don't set up shop. Work out of your
home and do talks to keep overhead down
until you've got a patient base. It wouldn't
fly to work from your home further south, but
Mainers prefer it. They don't want to pay
extra for the overhead. You would be
covered by insurance, so you'd have a leg
up on me. If you settle along the coast
within an hour of a fair-sized hospital you
should be fine.

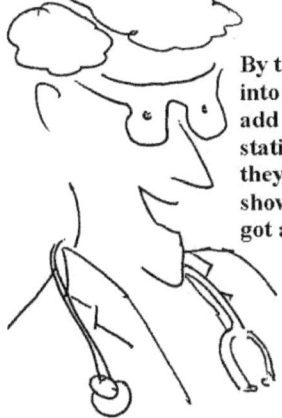

By the time a patient walks into my office, I know I can add 10% to his or her statistics. The simple fact they tracked me down and showed up means they've got a fighting spirit.

CHAPTER NINE: CHOOSING

Before you make your final choice, realize that there are people I try my hardest to convince not to take the N.D. route. If any of these ring familiar to you, be cautious about committing yourself.

People who I counsel against becoming N.D.s

Given how excited about the profession I am, there are still people I tell not to try it.

Here are a few pictures:

An older adult with a young, dependent family without other means of support. They will struggle through school with loans and still be trying to make ends meet for years after graduation.

A person who is already seriously ill and wants to get an N.D. degree for self-use. It's not a rewarding program for self-help. We get pushed a lot harder than someone with serious illness could handle. If you can't sit on your bottom for twelve hours of classes straight (yes, literally), think again.

A **professional who wants the degree because they want more respect** and a higher status within their current profession. Crossovers are usually suspect on both sides. I knew some great M.D.s in our program, but there were comments about them "stealing our medicine." Meanwhile, they got a lot of heat from their M.D. colleagues who thought they'd gone nuts. Having the second degree is wonderful for your patients, but plan to practice primarily Naturopathic medicine and to endure a great deal of skepticism from your colleagues.

Someone who thinks that becoming an N.D. will be easy. Often this person is considering a range of options including purchasing an online course. (Don't be surprised, you can also buy an M.D. diploma online). These people I generally redirect into one of the "highest" level of subfields, whether as

Christopher Maloney, N.D.

master herbalists or licensed massage practitioners or physical therapists.

I have much more respect for anyone who has undergone an in-person program with an experienced practitioner. Too often a diploma is just a piece of paper.

Like any medical school, naturopathic medical school will consume your life for four years. Outside of class time, there is research to conduct, papers to write, and hundreds of clinical hours of training.

Making your decision: Some tools.

The first thing I have many patients do when they are trying to make major life decisions is to **write down one hundred things they want to do** in their life. This reorients them away from one decision and refocuses them on the larger reality that this is just one aspect of their life. Please take the time to at least start the list now.

If most of the things you'd like to do involve money and prestige, you have your answer. If most of them involve you having extended time, you have another answer.

The second thing I make some patients do when they are confused about life is **write a statement of what they believe.** It's a useful exercise and can clarify for you if you are more likely to thrive in a large team or on your own.

The third project is to **turn your list of beliefs into a manifesto**, a paragraph or set of paragraphs that describe your belief structure.

Some of you won't find any of the above easy because it's difficult to clarify what you believe about some specific issues. Most of us hold a variety of beliefs about something rather than simply one. At times these beliefs are in direct conflict.

I condensed a book on decision-making into the following paragraph. Insert the word medicine for the important thing. Other good words would be: money, healing, family, and life.   By the way, **I don't like book exercises either. But this is a hundred thousand dollar, life-changing decision**. Take a few hours to make sure it's the right one.

SELF THERAPY

Pick something important to you (God, Money, Relationships, Time, **Medicine**, Health)

What is your first memory of this?
How did your parents experience it? What did they teach you?
What negative experiences have you had with this?
How is this holding you back in your life?

How do you move forward? (Problem
avoidance/goal setter?)

Write down twenty sentences about this.

(___is/are…)

What positive experiences have you had with this?

To what do you attribute those positive experiences?

Go back to your twenty sentences and rewrite them as
positive statements about you and your future.

Can you put all twenty sentences into a single
positive statement that will act as a goal?

Finally

You've made your decision. Now sit with
it overnight. Write yourself a letter explaining
to the future you why you are doing what
you're doing. You'll need this for the other
end, when it will be hard to remember why
you entered into this crazy medical world.

Christopher Maloney, N.D.

Will You Still Talk To Me If I Become an M.D.?

Absolutely. You might not talk to me. After years of medical training within the healthcare system, it is likely that you will resent me. Every time you spend all night in a hospital you might start to think: "and that guy thinks he's a doctor."

The model for becoming an M.D. is incredibly brutal. You will suffer at the hands of your brethren, and if you emerge with compassion and curiosity intact you have both my congratulations and my admiration.

But I will still be treating those patients unwilling to enter the medical model or who have been discarded by it. We would do well to talk to one another.

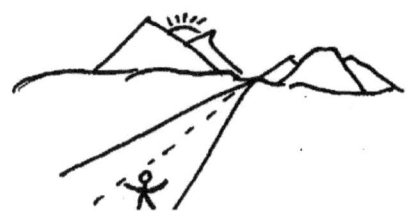

At the end, some things happen easily and some do not. If you feel like you are swimming upstream, change direction. Sometimes what we truly want needs to be achieved by taking the scenic route.

ABOUT THE AUTHOR

Christopher Maloney, N.D., graduated from Swarthmore College and completed his pre-medical studies at Harvard University. He graduated from the National College of Naturopathic Medicine (now the National College of Natural Medicine) in 2002, after completing a year's internship in Singapore and Malaysia. Dr. Maloney lives and practices in Augusta, Maine, where he divides his time between seeing patients, writing, and spending time with his wonderful family.

[i] Posted by Chris Maloney, ND on 12/22/02 at 08:34 PM at http://www.pandamedicine.com/rt_education/100-2.html

[ii] http://www.ncbi.nlm.nih.gov/pubmed/22017355

[iii] http://www.ncbi.nlm.nih.gov/pubmed/20354396

[iv] (http://www.quackwatch.org/01QuackeryRelatedTopics/reality.html).

[v] http://nprinstitute.org/outcomes-studies

[vi] http://www.ncbi.nlm.nih.gov/pubmed/12417803

[vii] http://humanbodyengineer.wordpress.com/tag/doctor-of-naturopathic-medicine/

[viii] http://www.pnhp.org/new_bankruptcy_study/Bankruptcy-2009.pdf

[ix] www.darmouthatlas.org. p.4, atlas and reports, Chronic illness atlas

[x] JAMA. 1998 Oct 14;280(14):1245-8.

[xi] JAMA. 2003 Jun 4;289(21):2849-56.

[xii] Mahar, Maggie. Money Driven Medicine. p. XV.

[xiii] Mahar, Maggie. Money Driven Medicine. p. XVI.

[xiv] Mahar, Maggie. Money Driven Medicine. p. XVI.

[xv] Mahar, Maggie. Money Driven Medicine. p.17.

[xvi] Mahar, Maggie. Money Driven Medicine. p.46.

[xvii] Mahar, Maggie. Money Driven Medicine. p.312.

[xviii] Mahar, Maggie. Money Driven Medicine. p.151.

[xix] http://en.wikipedia.org/wiki/Wilk_v._American_Medical_Association

[xx] Acad Med. 2009 Jun;84(6):707-11.

[xxi] http://www.shef.ac.uk/scharr/ir/percent.html